THE FUNCTIONAL MAMA

Federica Lippi

CONTENTS

A woman's body will change more in 9 moths of pregnancy than a man's will in his lifetime, and she needs an exercise program to match the transformation. A mom to be will need to master strength, agility, balance, speed, acceleration, deceleration, directional change and rotation, all with load that increases every day. For these reasons a "functional" fitness plan for an expectant woman may look different from a non-pregnant person's gym routine.

This guide helps new moms to comfortably perform the movements and tasks unique to a pregnant person, and how to be prepared for the birth experience and new role in a functional way.

CHAPTER 1
TRAINING FOR FUNCTION

"Functional training" means exercise designed to increase an individual's ability to carry out everyday tasks, that is, movement that mimics the real life tasks someone must carry out in an average day, such as repeatedly picking a baby up out of a crib or performing hobbies. These tasks are often described as activity of daily living.

Activity of daily living traditionally reference very basic activities, such as bathing, dressing, grooming, toileting and transferring(moving oneself about). However, a more comprehensive definition of "function" for an expectant mom might also include being able to work 8 hours a day, shop, cook, drive, and do housework, laundry and yard work. Certainly, there are medical conditions that preclude physical activity during pregnancy. Pregnant women should always obtain a medical opinion before starting a fitness program and seek ongoing input from a physician during training and listen to her bodỳs signals and slow down when needed. However, for women without medical complications, physical activity during pregnancy has been associated with important health benefits and should always be encouraged. The fact is that most of the pregnant women do not meet current recommended guidelines, they don't receive much diet and exercise counseling from their obstetricians. Therefore, this guide is on the frontline of wellness education for the need to know functional facts for moms to be.

CHAPTER 2
THE BIOMECHANICS OF PREGNANCY

The natural adaptive changes triggered by pregnancy may affect a woman's posture and biomechanics in the following ways:

Increased joint laxity
- during pregnancy, a woman's body produces more of the hormone relaxin, which "relaxes" ligaments (increases joint laxity), especially in the pelvis, hips and low back. This allows the female body to accommodate the growing uterus and, critically, prepares a woman to give birth vaginally. Relaxin production increases tenfold throughout pregnancy, peaking between week 38 and 42. This typically makes pregnant women noticeably more flexible than normal. Caution is advised during stretches.

Increases body weight
- a woman who begins her pregnancy at a normal weight will gain, on average, around 0.64 pounds of weight per week in her low trunk area. You should gain 25-35 pounds of weight overall at a rate of roughly one pound per week in the second and third trimesters.

This can make you less stable and more likely to lose your balance and fall, especially in later pregnancy.

Increase low back and pelvic pain

- the weight of your growing fetus may pull your pelvis forward into an anterior pelvic tilt (lordosis) and your growing breasts may create a kyphotic posture (shoulders rounded forward).

Postural changes

- to maintain good posture and be "functionally fit" you must be able to effectively recruit and use three important groups of muscular stabilizers:

1) the deep abdominals (transversus abdominals and internal obliques),

2) the hip abductors and rotators and

3) the scapular stabilizers

Yet pregnancy strongly impacts all these stabilizing muscles. As your belly grows, your abdominal muscles are gradually lengthened over your growing uterus, and the rectus abdominis muscles sometimes separate (a condition known as diastasis recti). In a mom to be, the abdominals lose tone, making you less able to effectively contribute to the maintenance of neutral posture. The hip stabilizes are also subject to unusual stressors. Physical adaptations of pregnancy are likely to place additional demand on hip abductors, hip extensors and ankle plantar flexors during walking.

CHAPTER 3
THREE FUNCTIONAL NEEDS OF PREGNANCY

The functional needs of an expectant woman are not static. They evolve along with the demands of nurturing her fetus and then her new baby. Consider the three impending "life events" for which you must train :

A new lifestyle:
Functional fitness must be customized. Are you going to work a physical or sedentary job during or/and after your pregnancy ? do you want to train for specific labor positions, such as a full squat ? do you have other small children whom you must carry around on the hip throughout your pregnancy? These are the kinds of real world concerns that must be factored into your functional exercise program.

Labor and Delivery:
Functional training for labor and delivery is akin to a sport specific protocol. This program focuses on preparing for birth in a manner similar to the way an athlete trains physically and mentally for a major competition. After all,

pregnant moms are likely to experience intense pain and muscular contractions during labor, all while possibly remaining awake for more than 24 hours

New Motherhood:

the demands of new motherhood must also be factored into your new pregnant fitness plan. Spend some time thinking through these demands, or watch a mom in your life as she moves through her world in a maternal role. You will start to see some much needed movement patterns to incorporate in your fitness training that will help you feel strong and possibly avoid injury

CHAPTER 4
FUNCTIONALTRAINING
FIRSTTIMESTER(WEEK1-12)
FOUNDATIONALCONCEPTS

Goals for early pregnancy

The key point during the first trimester is to help you ease into the tremendous shifts occurring in your body and prepare for the challenge the growing baby will put in your musculoskeletal system. At the outset of the first trimester, you should assess with a "primal movement" screen based on four key parameters, listed in order of functional importance:

1) core loading

2) hip loading

3) scapular loading

4) pectoral loading

For most pregnant women, the primary focus should remain on the hip loading and core/diaphragm/pelvic-floor activation. Scapular loading is the third priority, followed by all other concerns.

1) CORE LOADING (abdominals, diaphragm, pelvic floor)

The diaphragm is the functional component behind nearly all muscle imbalances. Proper diaphragmatic breathing is the single most important exercise for the modern pregnant woman. Our bodies have a physiologic response to deep breathing exercises. A result of this response is clarity in thinking and ease of muscular tension.

An example of a deep breathing exercise is "Diaphragmatic Breathing." Diaphragmatic Breathing not only reduces unwanted muscular tension, but also promotes core conditioning as it stretches and tones the diaphragm. The diaphragm is a muscle located at the top of the core (directly underneath the ribcage) and is primarily responsible for breathing. During pregnancy, the complex of breathing muscles comes under a surprising amount of stress. As baby grows, the diaphragm becomes compressed within the base of the ribcage, making breathing more difficult. To breathe, the body recruits muscles within the upper shoulders and back, making these muscles tight and contributing to a rounded (kyphotic) posture. The strategy for diaphragmatic breathing includes stretching the diaphragm to promote better breathing capabilities, better posture and a strong abdominal core!
Diaphragmatic Breathing is one of the essential factors for easing labor discomfort. Deep Breathing stimulates a parasympathetic response within the body, typically called

the "feel good response". It does so by stimulating a nerve within the diaphragm called the valgus nerve which helps release feel good hormones that: lower blood pressure lower heart rate,

increase blood supply to baby, create a sense of calm / peace within the body Furthermore, deep diaphragmatic breathing will help postpartum when the uterus needs to contract (involution) and return to its pre-pregnancy state.

Diaphragmatic Breathing exercise

Diaphragmatic Breathing Sitting Upright: Set-Up:

Sitting up-right (shoulders-over-hips), place one hand at the base of the ribcage and the other hand over the navel
Breath:
Inhale through the nose and purse the lips tight Exhale through the mouth, dropping the shoulders and releasing the lips
Inhale and as you deeply exhale notice the muscles underneath the bottom hand pulling the navel in, towards the front of the spine, and up, closer to the heart. Repeat, as you deeply exhale, notice the muscles underneath the top hand softening the ribcage back and scooping the belly under. As you continue breathing, notice the belly musculature underneath both hands narrowing the abdomen from the front, side and back. Remember to keep your inhalation gentle, meaning do not force the abdomen to expand (this may over stretch some of the superficial muscles). Repetitions and Timing: Begin with 3 breaths and "work-up" to ten. Postpartum women breathe in for 5 counts and exhale for 5 counts. Prenatal women breathe in for 2-5 counts and exhale for shorter duration 2-3 counts or 3-4 counts. During pregnancy the metabolism

changes so that you lose carbon dioxide more easily; this makes prenatal women more vulnerable to dizziness, nauseous and fainting.

Pelvic floor

Next, you should start incorporating pelvic-floor exercises in your first trimester. The earlier the training begins, the better. Gaining pelvic floor awareness is easier prior to introducing the load of a growing baby. Gaining and maintaining pelvis-floor strength will help prevent back and pelvic pain, incontinence and possible organ prolapse.

Pelvic floor exercises are an important part of your fitness program. The pelvic floor is a sling of muscles stretching across the floor of the pelvis. Attaching to your pubic bone at the front, the pelvic floor muscles stretch across the floor of your pelvis and attach to the coccyx (the tail at the end of your spine) at the back. Openings from your uterus, bladder and bowels all pass through your pelvic floor.

Here are some instructions and tips on how to perform excellent pelvic floor muscle exercises:

1) Try to keep the buttocks relaxed (sometimes these can squeeze involuntary as a way of keeping the pelvic floor lifted). Avoid clenching!
2) Make sure the muscles around your middle are relaxed and not contracted. Sucking in our tummies will also bear down on the pelvic floor, making it much more difficult or impossible to draw it up.

3)Breathe! The importance of breathing cannot be stressed enough! Holding your breath (probably because you are concentrating!) will bear down on the pelvic floor, even when you think you are pulling it up. Remember this tip for all exercises!

4) Start the contraction by pulling tightly closed the muscles around the back passage. Exactly like when you want to break wind in an inappropriate setting! And draw the pelvic floor up and to the front.

5) Allow the pelvic floor to descend back down. Always be aware when you are bearing down or straining on your pelvic floor and avoid this always.

6)Your pelvic floor is like any other muscle in your body: it needs different types of training for different uses. Practice your sprint exercises (quick, fast, grabby contractions)– these are handy for sneezes and coughs; but you also need to practice endurance—for the times when you need to hold on. These can be practiced by holding up your pelvic floor and counting slowly and being aware of how many seconds you can hold your pelvic floor up before you feel your buttocks clench, or you start holding your breath or it simply fades away. Working on your Personal Best and maintaining a hold of 8–10 seconds is a fantastic goal to work towards.

7)Your pelvic floor muscle responds really well to regular training, little by little —you can often feel improvement over just a few weeks. But unfortunately the opposite is also true: without practicing your exercises it can become weak again and cause you to leak again. These exercises are for life!

8) Your pelvic floor loves a challenge! Start to include it in your usual exercise routine. It may mean that you perform less reps and require much more concentration.

9) Your Grandmother loved you having good posture and

so does your pelvic floor. Holding your body upright will not only allow the pelvic floor to function better, but you will be able to breathe better, and in turn you will look and feel better! Posture counts as an exercise!

All of this information just might seem like too much hard work. But possessing a strong pelvic floor really can have some fantastic side effects. That flat belly that you have been lusting after since the birth of your child is achievable. Contracting the pelvic floor first will help contract those deep core muscles. A strong pelvic floor will increase your sexual satisfaction, giving you stronger orgasms and also increasing your partner's pleasure as well.

Finally, early pregnancy is also a great time to incorporate core-strengthening exercises. The first two exercises can be done prenatally, while the third can be added after baby arrives. You'll begin with the controlled movement of the sitting knee lift, which targets the spine-supporting abs and hip flexor muscles. The second exercise, the side-lying crunch, is especially useful after the fourth month of pregnancy, when women need to avoid performing exercises while on their backs. Finally, the bridging-with-a-curl move is great to incorporate in your postpartum routine.

PRENATALANDPOSTPARTUMEXERCISES

1. Sitting Knee Lift: Sit near the edge of a sturdy chair, feet flat on the floor directly under your knees. Place your hands, palms down, under your buttocks. Contract your abdominals to tilt your pelvis under; holding this position, bring your bent left knee toward your chest. Contract your abs further as you lower your left foot to the floor, using your abs to hold the position. Release the tilt to a neutral position and repeat. Do all reps with left leg, then repeat with the right. Do 2 sets of 8–12 reps in first trimester,
1–2 sets of 8–12 reps in second and third trimesters. During the first trimester, you can attach a 1- to 3-pound weight to each ankle for resistance. Strengthens abdominals and hip flexors.

2. Side-Lying Crunch: Lie on your left side, knees bent at a 30-degree angle to your hips. Roll over to the right only enough to lift your knees about 6 inches off the floor, your body weight resting on the back of your left shoulder and shoulder blade. Place both hands behind your head, fingertips touching but not clasped, elbows open. Curl torso up on the diagonal, bringing your breastbone toward your right knee. Your left shoulder will lift only slightly off the floor. At the top of the movement, reach both arms forward toward your knees, curling up a little higher. Place hands back behind head and lower to starting position, then repeat.
Do 1 set of 6 reps, then switch sides, progressing to 12 reps for all 3 trimesters.

Note: You probably should be able to perform this exercise comfortably into the beginning of your last trimester. If you have a diastasis, lift your torso directly upward, not on the diagonal. As your pregnancy progresses, and when you begin to exercise postpartum, help pull yourself upward by holding your thighs. You also can add a second set postpartum when the first is no longer challenging. Strengthens abdominals.

POST PARTUM ONLY

3. Bridging with a Curl: Lie face up on the floor with your heels on the seat of a chair, knees bent. Position yourself so your hips are about 6–8 inches behind your knees. Relax your arms by your sides. Keeping your lower back in contact with the floor, curl your torso upward, bringing ribs toward hips, until shoulder blades clear the floor. Holding this position, tilt your pelvis under, press down with your heels for leverage, and use your abs to lift your pelvis off the floor until your legs and hips form a straight line. Lower buttocks to the floor, then lower upper torso. Do 1 set of 8–12 reps; when that's comfortable, add a second set of 8 reps and build to 12 reps. Strengthens abdominals.

Suggestion: try it on Swiss ball for more stability strength.

2) HIP LOADING (Glutes, Low back)

As a new mom you're going to find yourself bending at the changing table, at the car seat and just about everywhere else until your kid is old enough to no longer be carried everywhere. The importance of a correct hip hinge technique education (loading the glutes) versus just rounding the spine when lifting, is crucial. Indeed, most pregnant women's glutes are under activated and deadlifts can improve this. However, a pregnant woman's back is significantly more at risk during unsupported forward flexion than when she is not pregnant, be caution !

For women who consistently struggle with deadlift technique, try a squat instead. Sumo squats are recommended, they support the sacroiliac joints as a woman's relaxin levels increase and her pelvis becomes increasingly unstable. When sumo squats are done correctly, the feet are about
6-10 inches wider than the shoulders, with toes turned out about 15 degrees. Progress both deadlifts and squats by holding a dumbbell at one shoulder in a manner that reflects how you will later be holding a newborn. Finally it is encouraged to try the deep squat position (knees and hips fully flexed, as if squatting to go to the bathroom outdoors) as labor and delivery training. This position creates the shortest and widest opening for the birth canal.

3/4) SCAPULAR & PECTORAL LOADING
(Midback,Chest)

It is very important to start strengthening the upper back and stretching the anterior chest muscles in order to combat the effects of gravity on a new mom. After all, you will soon spend hours rounding your shoulders forward to change, bathe, play and feed your new arrival. Work on strengthening the muscles of scapular retraction and include chest stretches. Suggested stretch is the doorway stretch (hands on each side of an open door, elbows back, body leans forward) several times a day. Also consider pushups.

As a mom to be, you're going to find yourself on the floor a lot, lying and playing with your newborn and emerging toddler. You are going to be performing one-sided and other strange varieties of pushing-up off the floor.

You must learn this pattern to be a functional mom !

FUNCTIONAL EXERCISES
FOR EARLY PREGNANCY
FIRST TRIMESTER EXERCISES

-squats, sumo or Swiss ball

-multidirectional lunges

-carry on (carry as heavy weight as you can for as long as you can with good posture)
-bent over row

-high and low cable pulls

- push ups

-wood chop

-balance exercises (eg. Bosu balance, balance board, Swiss ball)
-superman

-back extension

-exercises for the low abdomen

-pelvic floor exercises

-toe touch drill (balance one leg, slightly bent; touch other foot lightly to different cardinal points on the floor; pay attention to posture and knee tracking on the support leg)
-yoga poses (full squat held for 30-60 seconds, downward facing dog and cat cow, and breathing exercises to calm the min

CHAPTER 5
SECONDTRIMESTER(WEEKS 13-28)

Goals for mid pregnancy – the second trimester is when
you find that your energy level is returning and your "baby
bump" is starting to show. As a second trimester mom you
should begin building your strength and endurance in
preparation for baby weight gain.
At this stage, you should pay close attention on how an
exercise feels on the spine, abdomen and groin. When you
feel pulling or tightness, or just don't feel comfortable
anymore, you should discontinue that particular exercise.
Areas of importance include the core, the upper back and
the arms:

CORE STABILITY:

Concentrate on core strength in various planes of motion.
For example "the standing wood chop" is a highly
functional movement for moms. You should avoid lying
flat on your backs at this point in your pregnancy because
the baby weight of the growing baby could cause a relative
obstruction of venous return (it could impede the return
of blood from the lower body to the heart). This may

lower cardiac output and cause orthostatic hypotension (dizziness due to an acute drop in blood pressure). You can do modified supine (semi-sitting) or possibly, standing abdominal exercises for your core.

UPPER BACK AND ARMS:

The second trimester is the perfect time to focus on the upper body, as the postpartum period will encompass a lot of lifting. Start thinking through the load imbalance of motherhood. As a new mom you will hardly ever be equally loaded on both sided of your body, since you will often be carrying the baby in one arm for months to come. To compensate, use exercises that throw the body off just a little, such as low rows with one arm instead of two. Also include upper body movements that involve rotation and lever extension. For example : when a mom puts her baby in a crib, her arms are extended, she then rotated and flexes at the spine. Mimic some of that movement in a bicep curl plus a forward extension of the arms, with weights or tubing.

FUNCTIONAL EXERCISES
FOR MID PREGNANCY
SECOND TRIMESTER EXERCISES

-sumo squats

-toe-touch drill

-static or dynamic lunge

-seated row

-lateral pull down

-wood chop

-balance work

-increased arm work such as bicep curls and triceps extension

-pelvic floor work + add hip opening poses such as pigeon

-include light stretches and thoracic mobilizations with a foam roller, and stretch the abdominal area if needed.

CHAPTER 6
FUNCTIONALTRAINING
THIRDTRIMESTER(WEEKS29-40)

Goals for late pregnancy:

The third trimester is all about keeping exercising comfortably while maintaining fitness. This can take some skillful modification techniques. You will by now have high levels of relaxing in your system. For this reason, avoid quick changes of direction, especially laterally (eg. side lunges, wood chops), because the risk of ligamentous sprain increases.

Late trimester functional fitness should also address the upcoming birth event and anticipated postpartum activities of daily living.

Training for labor and delivery : to promote the muscular endurance needed during birth, it is encouraged to practice holding a pelvic floor contraction, a squat or an upright abdominal compression (pulling the bellybutton into the spine) for up to 90 second at a time. Learning to hold contractions for 90 seconds at a time will help tremendously during labor. You should also learn to consciously relax the pelvic floor after every contraction, as this will develop mind-body awareness and an ability to relax the pelvic floor during the pain of a labor contraction. Remember to think of birth positive mental imagery or phases during third trimester exercises.

Training for parenthood: Late pregnancy is a great time to learn about proper biomechanics for early motherhood. When reaching in and out of the car for groceries, or getting a child out of the crib or car seat, you should always find ways to perform the movements using your glutes, drawing your bellybutton in and protecting your back.

As a new mom you will spend many hours seated in a forward position while breast or bottle feeding. This practice is wonderful for bonding but hard on the mother's back. To mitigate this concern, you should be practicing strengthening exercises and thoracic mobilization moves you can do at home.

FOCUS ON FUNCTION

Training for a "functional fitness" during pregnancy means addressing both the postural and biomechanical shifts you will experience, as well as the impending events of birth and early motherhood. But the most important thing you can do is to pay attention to your body's signals and slow down when needed.

Exercise during pregnancy is to maintain the health of both mother and child and to prepare the body for birth, not to lose weight or get duper fit. As a pregnant mom you should talk to your doctor or midwife and be smart about your exercise goals.
As an expectant woman you should find a healthy balance between rest and exercise and remember it is a short time in the big picture. That is the fundamental truth of functional fitness during pregnancy.

"There is never a more important time than pregnancy to listen to your body"

EXERCISE WARNING SIGNS

If you experience any of these symptoms during a workout, stop immediately and refer to your doctor:

-vaginal bleeding

-dyspnea (shortness in breathing) prior to extension

-dizziness

-headache

-chest pain

-muscle weakness

-calf pain or swelling (this may be caused by thrombophlebitis i.e inflammation due to blood clots)

-preterm labor (uterine contractions)

-decreased fetal movement

-amniotic fluid leakage (a clear odorless fluid leaking from the vagina)

CHAPTER 7
POST-PARTUM SPECIALS

POST PARTUM SEX BASICS

As you settle into new motherhood, you might start thinking about getting busy in a way that doesn't involve changing diapers or feeding your newborn. For better sex after a baby, you'll want to strengthen your pelvic floor. Why is that so important? The strength of the pelvic floor contributes significantly to your sexual response, as well as the friction your partner experiences. Pregnancy typically weakens the pelvic floor due to hormonal changes, weight gain, pressure from the weight of the baby and stretching during labor and delivery.

A weakened pelvic floor can lead to incontinence, painful intercourse and a decrease in the intensity and frequency of orgasms. But the good news is that like any weakened muscle, the pelvic floor can be strengthened with exercise. The stronger your pelvic floor muscles are, the more blood flow you have to the area, which heightens sensitivity, and you'll also experience more intense contractions during orgasm.

EXERCISES
POST-PARTUM specials

Kegel exercises:

Kegel exercises are the best way to shape up your pelvic floor, but it's also important to strengthen your abdominals, hips and lower back, which is what this entire workout is designed to help you do. The workout can be done every other day. But remember that you must wait six weeks after delivery before starting; if you've had a Cesarean section, wait eight weeks and get your doctor's OK first

Your pelvic-floor muscles are the ones you use to stop the flow of urine. To do a Kegel, tighten those muscles for about 6 seconds, then release. Try to concentrate on just your pelvic-floor muscles and not the ones in your abs and buttocks. On days that you don't do this workout, try doing Kegels for 1 minute a few times a day.

Heel squeeze:

Lie facedown, resting your forehead on your hands, with your knees shoulder-width apart. Bend your knees so your feet are approximately 12 inches from the floor. Turn your toes out and bring your heels together..

Squeeze your buttocks as you press your heels together and do a Kegel. Hold for 2 counts, breathing normally, then release. Do 10 times; work up to 3 sets of 10.

Benefit: Strengthens glutes and deep hip muscles.

Leg Extension:

Get down on your hands and knees, with your wrists directly under your shoulders. Draw your abdominals up and in. Inhale, then exhale as you slowly extend your right leg straight back.

Hold for 2 counts as you do a Kegel. Keep your body still as you bring your right leg back to the starting position. Switch legs and repeat. Do 10 times on each side, working up to 3 sets of 10.

Benefit: Tones the transverse abdominis, the deepest abdominal muscle.

Bridge Squeeze:

Lie on your back with your knees bent and feet flat. Place a soft ball or pillow between your knees and draw your abdominals in. Inhale, then exhale as you tighten your buttocks and lift your hips until your body forms a straight line.
Squeeze the ball for 2 counts as you do a Kegel, then lower hips. Do 10 times; work up to 3 sets of 10.

Benefit: Strengthens abdominals.

LIVE FUNCTIONALLY
TRAIN FUNCTIONAL

www.ingramcontent.com/pod-product-compliance
Lightning Source LLC
Chambersburg PA
CBHW062030280526
45787CB00005B/2267